BETTER ANSWERS TO TOUGHER QUESTIONS!

Richard Leslie Parrott, Ph.D.
President and Founder, Seize Your Life, Inc.

Published by: *Seize Your Life, Inc.*

ISBN: 978-0-9754537-3-5

Dedication

This book is dedicated to an *individual* and a *group:*

To my friend and colleague, Doug Little, Ph.D.: together we helped scores of doctoral students find "better solutions to tougher problems."

To my "Sunday Evening Supper Group": where good friends, good food, and good conversation unearth the treasures of practical wisdom.

Table of Contents

Contents

You gain strength, courage, and confidence by every experience in which you really stop to look fear in the face. You are able to say to yourself, "I lived through this horror. I can take the next thing that comes along."
—Eleanor Roosevelt

Preface:
The Answer Is Inside You

I believe *the answer is inside you.* You are smarter than you think you are. You know a great deal about what is best for you and your situation.

This book presents a practical tool for embracing, increasing, and using your own inner wisdom. You can find better answers to your toughest questions. You can discover better solutions for your most difficult problems. The answer, the solution, is inside *you.*

You can help your teenager, coach a staff member, listen to a friend, and be a better spouse. The wisdom you need is inside you. It is contained in the raw ingredients of your personal experience. This book tells you how to transform your experience into practical wisdom, yielding better answers and solutions for your life

In the first three chapters you will learn that experience is a tough teacher. There are four questions that can transform your experience into valuable lessons and wise action. The questions help you and help you to help others.

Chapters four, five, and six describe why the questions work and why they might fail. Toxic relationships poison the "mental digestive system." This stops the flow of new understanding and insight.

Chapters seven through twelve outline the power of the questions when you enter a "human moment" with a safe person. To risk being real is the path to greater wisdom.

At the end of the book are six "T-N-T discussions" (*Think-N-Talk, Talk-N-Think*) you can use for personal reflection or with a group.

The four questions come out of my own experience of helping others discover their own answers and solutions. I have used the questions to guide people from all walks of life, facing all kinds of situations. When people feel safe enough to risk being real, the questions point the way to buried treasure, valuable gems of practical wisdom.

Great resources of personal wisdom reside within you. This little book may not improve your IQ. However, as you make these simple questions a habit you will increase your inner wisdom and practical good sense.

Richard L. Parrott, Ph.D.
October 5, 2006

The great questions are those an intelligent child
asks and, getting no answers, stops asking.
                                    —George Wald

CHAPTER 1

Experience Is the Teacher

Challenging situations, ripe with difficult questions, are all around. You need wise and practical answers.

- How can I help my children learn to make better choices?
- Why did my sales pitch work last time, but not this time?
- How can I help a staff member improve telephone skills?
- Why is my work-team struggling with so much conflict?
- How should my husband and I respond to this challenge?
- What is the best way to approach my new job?
- Why is the business doing so well right now?
- How can I help my friend who is in turmoil?
- What can I do to be more successful next time?
- Why is my boss so concerned about my performance?

1

- How will I explain this change to my team?
- What should I do next?
- Why did this happen to me?
- How will I ever get over it?
- What do I need to learn so I don't have to go through this again?

"I can't answer your questions right now!" blurts out a frustrated mother to her inquisitive three-year-old in the backseat. She balances driving the car, managing the errands, and carrying on a cell-phone conversation. The little one turns toward the window and swallows his desire to ask.

It is natural for children to ask questions about everything, all the time. A child is new to the world and trying to figure out what's happening and why. As an adult, your world is also full of new experiences:

Babies are born,
products change,
sales are up,
teenagers find trouble,
staff members need guidance,
customers are smarter,
the market shifts,
the marriage is strained,
the business expands,
sales are down,
civic duties call,
children leave home,
the promotion comes through,
a friend needs help,
the unexpected happens,
and on and on.

Life supplies a constant stream of opportunities and setbacks that demand sensible and practical answers. Each experience contains raw ingredients; facts and feelings, insights and understanding, learning and knowledge, options and actions.

The ingredients of practical wisdom and good answers fill your life like the ingredients of a meal fill a kitchen. Your task is to clean and chop, peel and dice, mix and stir, bake and boil, season and serve. A master chef transforms eggs, cream, and sugar into crème brûlée. You can transform your raw experiences into useful understanding and valuable wisdom.

The Components of Practical Wisdom

I was still reeling from a painful experience that carried all the components of potential wisdom. The loss of my position challenged personal identity. Relationships changed when friends stopped calling. My character was tested as I stood with integrity while others chose lower paths. It was a time of questioning purpose and meaning.

It was tempting to wallow in the hurt and "get stuck" in a pattern of self-pity. It is a path that leads to a personal prison of misery. Constantly rehashing the past, spewing out resentment against others, and playing the part of a victim are symptoms of a person who has never unearthed the wisdom in experience. I refused this path.

I determined that my experience would be transformed into something of value, something that would strengthen my resolve to be true to my best self. I took on the hard work of figuring out what had happened, exploring dynamics found below the surface of the situation, discerning lessons to be learned, and taking positive steps that helped me grow in authenticity and effectiveness.

Transform Experience into Answers

The experience just described was painful and confusing. However, other experiences are bright and hopeful. Still others are mundane and routine. Your experience is a great teacher. The lessons may be profound or simple, life changing, or just plain useful. But all experience, to be of value, must be transformed into practical answers and positive solutions.

This book presents a simple recipe for finding your own answers and cultivating your inner wisdom. Four questions, asked in the right order and with an open mind, lead to amazing answers. The message of this book is simple:

> Ask the right questions
> in the right way
> and you help yourself and others
> find better solutions
> to life's tougher problems.

The recipe, just four questions, works at the office, back home, in the board room, or over dinner. As you learn to ask yourself these questions, you will find that you are helping yourself. They will help you gather information, discover insights, learn, and act. With a little practice, you will soon unearth better answers to perplexing problems.

The questions are also a tool for helping others. You can encourage friends, mentor colleagues, coach staff members, and teach children to think for themselves. In a short while, the questions will no longer be a recipe to follow, but a habit that empowers your ability to guide others.

Experience IS the Teacher

Some things can only be learned through experience. You cannot learn to swim unless you get in the water. The same is true for relationships, parenting, leadership, counseling, teaching, sales, management, and all the arts and professions.

The room was full of students eager to begin their doctoral studies in leadership. As their professor, I previewed the course, the requirements, and the readings. I then asked them if they had brought their textbooks with them to class. They held up the books they had purchased at the university book store.

I insisted that I didn't see the "large textbook." I told them, "It's the one you will refer to most often. It is a costly book. And, without it, the class will be meaningless."

Their look of consternation lingered for a few moments. When attention was focused, I made my point, "The most important textbook is your personal experience. You will develop wisdom as you master the art of thinking about your own experience and the experience of others."

The most important life lessons are learned from experience. This is true for those who lead others. It is also true for parents, marriage partners, friends, and everyone who seeks more meaning and significance in life.

The art of thinking about your experience is the way to increase your inner wisdom. However, when you don't seek out the wisdom in your experience, you run the risk of falling onto a treadmill of dysfunctional ruts and routines.

The old story of "trimming the ham at both ends" illustrates the point. A young bride wanted to cook a ham for her husband. She called her mother and asked for help. Mom said, "First, trim a little off both ends of the ham before you put it in the roasting pan."

The young woman heard the advice, but something seemed amiss. She asked her mother why she trimmed the ends off the ham. Her mother said with confidence, "Your grandmother always trimmed the ends off the ham. I learned by watching her."

Now, the young bride was intrigued. She called her grandmother and asked about trimming both ends of the ham. Grandmother replied that she learned this trick by watching great-grandmother.

Fortunately, great-grandmother was still living. When she was asked the same question, the lovely old woman giggled as she reveled the secret, "Oh, my dear, I trimmed the ends of the ham because my roasting pan was too small."

The Right Questions

Good teachers assign homework. Experience is no exception. Assignments come in the form of headwork and heart work. Learning from experience is both rational and emotional. It takes facts and feelings.

Ask the right questions, in the right way, and you engage both head and heart. That's when you find the best answers, the wise answers. This book is about doing just that.

You will learn the four questions. Use all four questions. The questions help you (and help you to help others) dig below the surface of a problem to discover buried treasure—the practical answers you need.

You will learn what it means to be a "safe person." Intimidation, control, and blame shut down learning. That's when people fall into the cycle of doing the same thing, but hoping for different results. You can help people feel safe enough to question what's being done and look for new answers.

When you risk being real, the right questions will transform experience into practical wisdom. You are smarter than you think. This book provides a simple way to help you realize how much you already know and enhance your potential to learn so much more.

Find the right questions. You don't invent the answers, you reveal the answers.

—Jonas Salk

CHAPTER 2

The Four Questions

For thirty years I have been helping individuals and organizations find answers by asking the right questions. Over those years, I have had many roles: minister of a large congregation, professor at a university, director of a doctoral program, executive director of a leadership center, corporate trainer, organizational consultant, husband, father, and friend.

In each role I have found that asking the right questions in the right way is essential to my own success and the success of others. For years, I attempted to create new questions for each situation. The result was confusion and frustration. What I needed was a pattern of questions, a model or recipe that works in diverse situations.

Over time, through my academic studies, trial and error, and multiple revisions, I developed a gourmet recipe of four questions that are effective in the majority of situations and challenges people face. They form a pattern for analyzing your successes and learning from your regrets.

The questions provide a plan to solve problems, make team decisions, and understand complex issues. You can use them to work through conflict, conduct an interview, or coach a colleague. They help you guide others toward better solutions and answers.

The same questions will also guide your personal search for insight and meaning. Your thoughts and emotions form your inner experience. The wisdom you discover here is essential to staying true to your best self. The questions aid your quest for authenticity and effectiveness.

THE FOUR QUESTIONS

1.
What is happening?

2.
What is causing it to happen that way?

3.
What can I learn?

4.
What will I do next?

The questions open a path of self-discovery for you and for others. After seventy years, *How to Win Friends and Influence People* by Dale Carnegie continues to be published and purchased. One sentence Dale Carnegie wrote summarizes the challenge of the four questions: "An effective **leader** . . . will ask questions instead of giving direct orders." (See *How to Win Friends and Influence People*; Pocket Reissue edition 1990)

The Four Questions

Adapt and apply Carnegie's thought. Look over the list below. When you find a role that is yours, read the statement slowly. Imagine the impact of shifting your approach from giving answers to asking questions:

An effective **mother**	will ask questions instead of giving answers.
An effective **father**	will ask questions instead of giving answers.
An effective **wife**	will ask questions instead of giving answers.
An effective **husband**	will ask questions instead of giving answers.
An effective **supervisor**	will ask questions instead of giving answers.
An effective **mentor**	will ask questions instead of giving answers.
An effective **coach**	will ask questions instead of giving answers.
An effective **teacher**	will ask questions instead of giving answers.
An effective **counselor**	will ask questions instead of giving answers.
An effective **minister**	will ask questions instead of giving answers.
An effective **friend**	will ask questions instead of giving answers.

I had just finished teaching the four questions at a seminar. Returning to our room, my wife, Shirley, commented, "You use those questions with me all the time."

For us, the questions are a habit of heart and mind. They provide a way for us to tackle problems. They help us work together, appreciate one another's perspectives, and find better solutions. It is a way of talking together that is respectful, inquisitive, and that honors one another.

A Habit of Productive Thinking

The questions create a habit of productive thinking and healthy interaction. Each question pushes toward personal responsibility and mutual respect:

- **What is happening?** The question challenges you to take stock of your outward actions and observations as well as your inward thoughts and feelings. Begin with the way things are rather than the way you wish they were.
- **What is causing it to happen that way?** Complex problems have multiple causes. This question moves you from blaming to understanding, from jumping on easy explanations to exploring deeper dynamics.
- **What can I learn?** The question challenges you to learn if you have been part of the problem and how you can be part of the solution. In most complex situations, everyone has played a role in creating the problem, and it will take everyone to implement a good solution.
- **What will I do next?** Rather than waiting for everyone else to change, you can lead the way by changing what you do and how you respond. You

can take positive action that will help others envision a better way.

Applying the four questions is not a technique to gain power and control over others. It is not a method to manipulate or hoodwink people. If you seek useful answers, you must engage in authentic, healthy relationships. The questions work when interactions are healthy; when you relate to others with genuine and appropriate empathy, acceptance, transparency and boundaries. The best answers and most valuable solutions are revealed when individuals are authentic with one another. The result is productive thinking.

Establish Communication and Build Trust

It was a great opportunity for positive change. It was also a battlefield of hidden landmines. The "movers and shakers" in government and business, in city and county were willing to meet. The group had never had a joint meeting. The level of tension was high. Resentments ran deep. Hope of cooperation was a faint flicker at best.

The meeting marked the beginning of a new way government and business leaders would work together. In time, supportive and joint initiatives for the economic development of the city and county became the norm. Five years after this initial meeting, the editor of the local paper remembered the event in the following editorial:

> The cooperative and collaborative efforts between
> local government and business officials that have become
> a hallmark of Ashland's economic development effort are

a relatively new phenomenon in Ashland County. They have become so commonplace it's easy to take them for granted. However, I had forgotten this latest incarnation of local economic development had its real roots in a series of informal discussions initiated in 2000 . . . (*Ashland Times-Gazette*, February 24, 2005)

I had been asked to facilitate these initial "informal discussions." The meeting took place in the president's dining room at the university where I was employed. Representatives of county and city government, economic development groups, and the chamber of commerce attended.

The agenda items were apparent: exchange strategic plans, clear the air, learn to work together, and agree on the next step. But what would be the best way to transform this group of competitors into a coalition for the greater good?

I used the four questions to outline the meeting. First, to get at **what is happening** now, each group wrote is vision/purpose statement and major goals on individual flip charts. Then, each participant moved freely around the room, reading the statements, and noting items that could be a source of potential conflict or cooperation.

The lights came on. It was apparent that overlapping agendas and lack of communication contributed to ongoing turf struggles and misunderstandings. Of course, there was more to it than that. To reveal **what is causing it to happen that way** included unearthing personal issues, unresolved conflicts, and years of mistrust.

The conversation was heated. Yet, everyone stayed with it, sharing an unspoken understanding that this was the moment for change. A role play with a realistic issue allowed participants to see the dynamics and causes of cooperation and conflict. It helped them clarify **what we can learn** about working together.

Open and courageous communication, dealing with facts rather than rumor or suspicion, giving individuals time and space to wrestle with decisions, and seeking internal commitment to change were key lessons. The "wisdom" that came out of the meeting became practical as the group discussed **what we will do next.**

The action plan included a second meeting with wider participation. This was followed by changes in personnel in a few of the key organizations. A task group continued to meet and communicate with everyone involved. Eventually city- and county-wide meetings were held.

If you ask those who have been part of the process from the beginning, they will tell you it is a new day. This diverse group of individuals and organizations from a small city and the surrounding county found a better solution to a tough problem.

The editorial, written a half decade later, remembered the success of the:

> "informal discussions . . . to establish communication and build trust among community leaders. The focus of that dialogue shifted to improving economic development efforts, from which came the current initiatives. Such cooperation wasn't always the case on the local scene."

The important thing is to not stop asking questions.
—Albert Einstein

CHAPTER 3

The Four Questions Work!

Peter Drucker, in *The Effective Executive,* notes the difference between "doing things right" and "doing the right thing." The first is efficiency and the second is effectiveness. "Doing the right thing" (being effective) is the more important challenge. (See *The Effective Executive,* Revised, Harper Business, 2002)

When you find yourself in a situation that presents clear direction and tested routines, you should focus on efficiency or "doing things right." However, when the state of affairs is confusing and uncertain, your priority must be to determine an effective solution, the "right thing" to do.

When you want to maintain *efficiency,* give people answers.
When you need to discover what's *effective,* ask questions.

When you give answers, you appear competent, well-organized, capable, proficient, resourceful, and professional. It is an efficient use of time and a demonstration of ability to "give the answer." However, it is not always the most effective way to help others.

On occasion, when leading a group, I am asked a question that needs an immediate and efficient answer. These are questions that deal with facts or clarification. At other times, the questions are more complex and personal. In this case, providing an on-the-spot answer is not an effective approach. People learn more if they discover an answer personally.

Personal Discovery

A participant in one of my leadership development seminars asked a complex question concerning his office and staff. Rather than providing an expected and ready-made answer, I responded by asking him the four questions:

- *What is happening?* He assumed I needed more information before I gave him the answer. He unfolded the details. I pulled out additional facts with a simple follow-up remark, "And what else?"
- *What is causing it to happen that way?* This question surprised him. He expected me to tell him what to do next, now that he had given me the information. My question on "cause" pushed him to think for himself. Forty people were listening to this exchange. Of the forty, I knew he was the most knowledgeable on the situation; it was his office.
- *What can you learn?* He was confused. No one had ever asked that before. Like a school child, he struggled to come up what he thought I would accept as the "right" answer. I didn't want a "right" answer for me. He needed a wise answer for himself.

- *What will you do next?* Now, he was at a loss. That was what he wanted me to tell him. I was not living up to his expectations. Rather than think it through, he was asking for someone to tell him what to do.

It was apparent he was frustrated. I wrote out the four questions and challenged him to keep digging for his own answer. We didn't speak about the incident for almost a year. By then, a friendship had developed between us. We were enjoying a holiday meal together when he reminded me of our exchange at the seminar. He said,

> *When I asked you my question, I expected you to give me the answer. It was frustrating when you put the question right back on me. I didn't understand why you did it, and I didn't like it. But now I get it. When I discover the answer, I really know it.*

He had been learning to use the questions at home, at the office, and even in his responsibilities on the hospital board. He shared stories of how the questions had helped a staff member, solved a problem at the hospital, and opened communication at home. The questions are effective. They work!

Inner Confidence

Let me make one more observation: my friend's inner confidence has increased. He is learning to mine the resources of inner wisdom. He is learning that he is smarter than he thinks. He has discovered how to find better answers to tougher problems.

It is tempting to hold to the false hope that the "golden key" resides in the latest book, the next seminar, or with the most popular expert. It doesn't. The "golden key" is you. What you learn from experience and the experience of others is stored in a great reservoir of inner wisdom that lives within you.

In a culture that gives answers through every advertisement, family expert, and management guru, it is tempting to stop thinking for yourself. The four questions will sharpen and clarify your thinking. You will surprise yourself as you come up with wise answers that work.

Learning is the essential fuel for the leader, the source of high-octane energy that keeps up the momentum by continually sparking new understanding, new ideas, and new challenges. It is absolutely indispensable under today's conditions of rapid change and complexity. Very simply, those who do not learn do not long survive as leaders.
                              —Warren Bennis and Burt Nanus

CHAPTER 4

Use ALL Four Questions

The vast and empty desert of Namibia in Southwest Africa contains the diamond fields. They say that the diamonds are lying on the surface. I don't know if this is true. I have crossed Namibia in a Land Rover. We stayed away from the diamond fields. It is forbidden to enter the area. The guard patrols are ordered to shoot first and ask later.

Diamonds, like valuable insights and answers, are not often found on the surface. They are buried. You have to dig them out. That's the purpose of the four questions. They are tools for mining what is hidden, covered, or obscure. They help you (and help you to help others) get at the deeper problem, the murky issue, the unclear situation, and the answers that are more difficult to unearth.

Easy answers are everywhere. They may not be the right or best answer, but they are found on the surface of things. Here is how you gather them up: Ask the first of the four questions, and then jump to the last:

1. What is happening?
2.
3.
4. What will you do next?

Alone, these two questions work like a garden rake: they drag in what's lying around on the surface—what you've done before, what is obvious (but not always the best), what is expected, and what you can do without much thinking. This will get you through the day. It might even get you through a crisis. But it will not produce the breakthrough you need.

It is the middle questions (questions 2 and 3) that form the pick and shovel of new thinking. Together with questions 1 and 4, they become the tools that excavate fresh answers:

1. What is happening?
2. What is causing it to happen that way?
3. What can you learn?
4. What will you do next?

It takes more effort to use a pick and shovel than to use a garden rake. It takes deeper and better thinking to work through *all* of the questions. Deeper thinking gets at better answers. It also helps you develop professionally and personally. It helps you help others improve at what they do and increase their personal confidence.

Stop and Work on the Resistance

In my role as a professor, I incorporated the current experience of students in the classroom. One incident involved a course in group dynamics. The entire division of the graduate school was on the verge of a profound change.

A shift in curriculum was about to transform the master's program by implementing small study and support groups. The change had been adopted by the faculty and would be implemented the next semester.

I wanted students in the group dynamics class to design the new study and support groups as their major assignment. I felt rather clever and satisfied with my innovative approach. The students' current experience would be integrated into their education.

However, my *personal* experience in the first session of the course changed my plans and challenged me to search for practical wisdom. My suspicions were aroused when the students accepted the assignment in complete silence, no questions at all. I had to find out "what's happening."

It didn't take long to gather facts and feelings. The students were dead set against the curriculum change. I quickly went through the four questions in my own mind. I had a problem and needed the wisdom to know what to do next. It was time to stop and work on their resistance to the curriculum change or the resistance would stop the work of the class.

My first challenge was to transform a silent classroom into a safe place to discuss real problems and conflicts. The students needed to hear from me that this was the right time to work on the project, and they were essential to its success.

They also needed to know that I wanted what was best for them, rather than just to use them to implement a plan for the curriculum committee. Finally, they needed to hear from me, "When we are true to what is best in us, we will discover the best solution."

I went on to say, "We are all human beings attempting to deal with change. Let's learn from each other and see if we can make a positive difference." I then guided them through the questions.

- **What's happening?** Each person wrote multiple answers on separate post-it notes. We stuck all of them on the white board. The group sorted, discussed, and cataloged them into several groupings.
- **What is causing it to happen that way?** The usual suspects were rounded up: lack of communication, time pressure, fear of the unknown, and feeling overlooked and overworked.
- **What can you learn?** They needed help with this question. I rephrased it, "What will be the result if students continue resisting the impending change?" Examining their potential loss, academically and personally, increased their sense of responsibility and their desire to do something positive.
- **What will you do next?** I had barely gotten the question out before they were making action plans. They decided to visit the dean, professors, and other students. They determined to understand the change and make it work for the good of their education.

As a result of their actions, they embraced the change and helped other students to see the benefits. And, they put their whole hearts and minds into the assignment of designing small support and study groups.

Nine weeks later, this same group of students held a seminar for all the professors in the department. They outlined the design and purpose of the small groups that would soon be implemented. One of the students in the class was immediately hired by the dean's office to oversee the small groups for the next two years.

The questions help you (and help you help others) grapple with tough issues, air concerns, deal with facts, and make an internal commitment to change.

. . . that is what learning is. You suddenly understand something you've understood all your life, but in a new way.

—Doris Lessing

CHAPTER 5

Why the Questions Work

How can the same questions work in different situations with different people? I have had great success using the questions with children and adults. I know the questions work at home as well as on the job. They are helpful in a marriage, a family, a business, a church, a department, or any organization.

- The questions work in complex situations that demand better answers.
- The questions work when relationships are healthy and strong.
- The questions work with individuals who are authentic and genuine.
- The questions work for people who are willing and ready to learn.

More than forty years ago, Harvard Professor David Kolb began to explore why people learn best from personal experience. His theory of learning continues as a foundation stone for the best practices in both education and leadership.

(See *Experiential Learning: Experience as the Source of Learning and Development,* Financial Times, Prentice Hall, 1983)

Yet, experience is not the same as learning. You've heard it said, "He has thirty years of experience." If the truth were known, he may have three years of experience, ten times over. Experience must be transformed into wisdom. It is a process, like digestion.

Mental Digestion

Imagine that your personal experience (a success or regret) is a nutritious meal you have just devoured. You have taken in facts, thoughts, feelings, and intuitions, like swallowing meat, potatoes, vegetables, and a scrumptious dessert. The experience is inside you, just as the food is in your stomach.

Your mind must now start a process that turns experience into wisdom just as your body begins the process that turns food into energy. The process of digestion transforms the meal in your stomach into healthy energy for your body. Without digestion, you would continue eating while you starve to death.

There is a process of mental digestion that turns experience into wisdom. Your experience is in your mind. It contains the knowledge, learning, and wisdom you need. Your successes and regrets are filled with insights, ideas, and understanding that have the potential to energize better answers and actions.

You need to digest your experience. You must chew on it, break it down, put it together in new forms, and absorb what is helpful. The four questions engage and guide your mental digestive system.

Four Ways to Learn

Professor Kolb helped me understand how the mental digestive system works. He cataloged the different ways people learn. He discovered that there are two ways people receive new learning: by *experience* and by *thinking.* He also found that there are two ways people process new learning: by *watching* and by *action.*

Here's my way of presenting Dr. Kolb's theory in everyday language:

- Learning begins with *experience*—you rely on your senses, feelings, intuition, and personal involvement to know what is happening.
- Learning continues with *watching*—you observe, listen, consider other viewpoints, and make careful judgments about underlying dynamics, motives, and origins inherent in the situation.
- Learning then moves to *thinking*—you use your own logic, develop your own theories, and calculate the reasons of mind and heart as you determine what you can learn from the situation.
- Learning is put to the test in *action*—you focus on what's practical, what works, and what needs to be done, as you respond to the situation with plans and openness to new potential.

The Four Ways People Learn

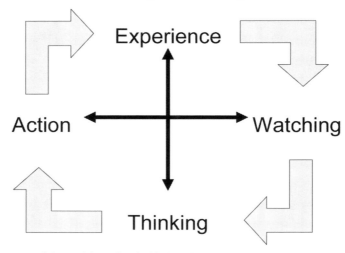

Adapted from David Kolb's *Experiential Learning*

The best learning comes when you use all four: experience, watching, thinking, and action. The four questions utilize all the ways people learn.

- The first question helps you sort out your own experience by asking, what happened? Consider the outside and inside of your experience. Note your observations and actions as well as your thoughts and emotions.
- The second question causes you to look for patterns by asking, what is causing it to happen that way? Patterns are discovered by compiling the facts as will as by exploring a hunch. Depend on accuracy and imagination.

- The third question pushes you to think beyond the situation by asking, what can I learn? Learning comes as your mind calculates consequences and conclusions. Learning also comes from the heart, which has its own source of wisdom.
- The fourth question moves you to test what you have learned by asking, what will I do next? Action plans form a tenuous agreement between solid decisions and openness to new possibilities.

The Four Questions

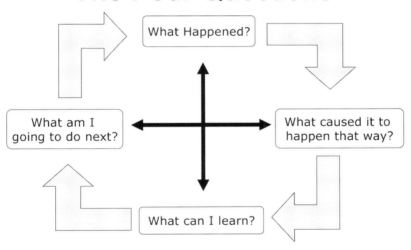

Developed by Richard L. Parrott

The questions work because they activate your mental digestive system. They do not provide answers. They get your juices churning so you can discover your own answers.

You have heard the saying Experience is life's greatest teacher. But experience alone cannot teach. You must sort out your experience (what's happening?), find the underlying patterns and dynamics (what's causing it to happen that way?), discern the lessons (what can I learn?), and use the energy (what will I do next?) to face the next challenge.

If you do not ask what it is you know, you will act on what you hear from others and deep change will not come because you will not hear your own truth.
—Saint Bartholomew

CHAPTER 6

Personality and the Four Questions

You have preferences. You prefer some styles of music over others. You have preferences for certain forms of entertainment or ethnic foods. On occasion, you listen to other styles of music or go to dinner at a restaurant that is not your first choice. Preferences don't have to limit life, but they do predict your inclinations.

Your personality is made up of preferences. You may prefer to make a decision and stick to it, or you may be more comfortable staying open to what comes next. At the end of a demanding day, some people are rejuvenated by exercise or going out with friends. Others find that a little quiet time alone is invigorating.

Personality preferences impact the way individuals utilize the four questions. Some people search for all the pieces of their experience. When they pile the parts together, they understand what is happening. Others start with a gut feeling and check it out to see if it's true.

Your personality has a preferred way to seek better answers and solutions. Your preference helps you make the most of each question, just as being right- or left-handed determines the best way to pick up a tool.

First, you can appreciate and use your preferences once you understand them. Preferences are not good and bad, just comfortable. It is almost always best to first approach a problem in a way that feels normal and natural to you.

Second, you can seek the help of people who have a different approach to solving problems. Approaching a problem in another way uncovers additional insight.

Third, you can learn different ways to think, ways you may not prefer at first. Learning to think in a different way, to tackle a problem with another approach, is challenging. However, the reward for your effort will be deeper and more practical wisdom.

There are two preferences for each of the four questions. You use both preferences just as you use both of your hands, right and left. However, most people find that one preference is stronger than the other.

Question One: "What is happening?"

"Look Out" and "Look In"

The first question is an examination of experience, a look at what is happening. Every experience has an inside and outside. Part of your experience is what is going on around you. The other part is what is happening on the inside.

"Look Out"—focus on the outside; people, events, and actions. They center attention on what they see and what they do.

"**Look In**"—focus on the inside; reflection and contemplation. They center attention on what they think and what they feel.

In order to explore the whole experience, you need both, the outside and the inside. You also have a preference for starting with one or the other. Start with your preference, but continue to explore the other side.

Answer What is happening? by noting the following:

- What I saw.
- What I did.
- What I thought.
- What I felt.

Question Two: "What is causing it to happen that way?"

"See the Trees" and "See the Forest"

The second question is a search for dynamics and patterns, a hunt for what is causing things to happen this way. There are two ways to search for causes. You can sift through the details or you can step back and get a big picture of what is happening. It takes both, the trees and the forest.

"**See the Trees**"—consider the details with precision. Consider each tree in the forest. Collect the specifics accurately. Follow the facts to the cause.

"**See the forest**"—summarize and use your imagination. Look at the forest as a whole. Imagine the possibilities. Follow your insights and hunches.

In order to understand hidden causes, you need both, the trees and the forest. You will begin with the one you prefer, but you need to develop the opposite approach also.

Answer What is causing it to happen that way? by reflecting in the following way:

- Look at the details.
- Check their accuracy.
- Summarize them.
- Imagine possibilities.

Question Three: "What can I learn?"

"Head First" and "Heart First"

The third question is a challenge to unearth a nugget of wisdom, to express what you can learn from what is happening. People approach a mental challenge either head first or heart first. There is wisdom derived from reason. There is also the wisdom of the heart.

"Head First"—use logical reasoning to arrive at underlying principles. Being rational is one way to face the challenge of producing a gem of wisdom.

"Heart First"—discover the wisdom revealed by exploring significant value and relationships. The heart has wisdom rational calculations cannot discover.

In order to mine the wealth of wisdom in your experience, you need both head and heart. Begin with what is natural for you, head or heart. Then, challenge yourself to search again with the opposite method, heart or head.

Answer the question, What can I learn? by searching for the following:

- The logical conclusions.
- The rational principles.
- The significant values.
- The impact on people.

Question Four: "What will I do next?"

"Finishers" and "Starters"

Question four is an application of the practical wisdom you have discerned in the first three questions. Some people turn wisdom into action as a finished product. Others view the action that comes from wisdom as starting a new process. It is both, the finishing line and the starting gate.

"Finishers"—make a decision and stick to the plan. Applying practical wisdom means getting things done, having things settled, and following plans through to the end. It often involves schedules and specific tasks.

"Starters"—look for options and don't be hemmed in by prior decisions. Apply your wisdom by looking for better alternatives, staying open to new possibilities, and facing challenges as they come along.

Applying your practical wisdom is choosing what to do next. It is both a finished product and the start of a process. It is deciding on a plan and staying open to better possibilities. It is staying true to your decision, but not being hampered by it.

Answer, What will I do next? by doing the following:

- Decide on a plan.
- Follow the plan.
- Stay open to options.
- Tackle what comes.

Have you determined your preferences? Remember, everyone utilizes all the preferences at one time or another. Appreciate your preferences, your style of solving problems and finding answers. Seek the help of people who have a different style.

Finally, challenge yourself to answer the four questions using ALL the preferences. You will find better answers to your toughest questions.

There are people who learn, who are open to what happens around them, who listen, who hear the lessons. When they do something stupid, they don't do it again. And when they see something that works a little bit, they do it even better and harder the next time. The question to ask is not whether you are a success or a failure, but whether you are a learner or a nonlearner.
—Benjamin Barber

C H A P T E R 7

Why the Questions Could Fail

Magicians keep their secrets. To expose them would destroy the magic. Hidden panels, sleight of hand, audience distractions, and carefully crafted items are locked away from public view. To share the secret or reveal the trick would ruin the illusion. The magic would vanish.

In the *Wizard of Oz,* the frightening image of the "Great and Powerful Oz" is shattered in a moment when Toto parts the curtain revealing the source of the fantasy. "Pay no attention to that man . . ." are useless words. The secret is out. The curtain on the four questions will now part. Pay close attention. Here is the magic:

The questions work when you feel safe enough to risk being real.

When you risk being real, you are more open and aware of the internal and external dimensions of your experience. When you feel psychologically safe, you are more apt to consider alternative explanations and insights. Greater wisdom emerges from personal honesty and courageous authenticity. When you feel safe, you risk being real and the questions work.

Questions are Uncomfortable

Yet, questions mean danger to most people. When someone asks questions, you could be in jeopardy. The three-year-old in the back seat of the car hears mother scold, "I can't answer your questions now." In a little while, the child will learn it is best to stop asking questions.

A few years later, in grade school, the child may learn that it is best to avoid questions altogether. Let others answer. After all, if you answer incorrectly, you might be teased. And, if you answer correctly, you might be labeled "teacher's pet" or a "show off."

Think of the times when questions are a sign of danger:

Who broke the window?
The test questions will determine your grade.
Why isn't the report on my desk?
The screening consists of seventy questions.
Are you going to meet quota this month?
I have a few questions concerning your tax return.
When are you going to get it right?
If you answer correctly, you have nothing to worry about.
Whose fault is it?

People are talking; they have serious questions.
Are you on target with your assignment?

In many organizations, it is imprudent to question the boss. It is a sign of impending disaster if the outside consultant asks you to "answer a few questions." In the family, on the job, or by the government, being questioned is often a fearful experience. You are put on the spot. Your weakness is exposed. Someone will be blamed, and you don't want to be tagged.

Fear will negate the magic of the four questions. The questions are designed to uncover better answers and deeper insights. However, when people are afraid, they will cover, hide, and distort. In a fearful atmosphere, the questions will not function.

Fear Poisons Relationships

Fear is the first indication of toxic relationships. When families or organizations operate with hidden motives and agendas, insensitivity and indifference, an emotional poison runs through the system. Pain is part of life, but when painful situations are handled in cruel or heartless ways, better answers and wise solutions are the first casualties.

WHEN RELATIONSHIPS ARE TOXIC:
The questions may intimidate and coerce.

- *What is happening?* An automatic censor takes over to screen out potentially dangerous facts and cover vulnerable emotions.

- *What is causing it to happen this way?* The question becomes a race to place blame and protect vested interests.
- *What can you learn?* The response will be designed to meet expectations and give the appearance of personal competence.
- *What will you do next?* Individuals choose a strategy that gets them out of danger and safeguards them from facing it again.

Toxic relationships carry a "fear virus" that shifts mental energy toward self-protection and escape. The inner wisdom buried in individuals, teams, and the experience lies dormant.

Because "being questioned" is often associated with fearful emotions, do everything possible to lower the lever of apprehension. Work to eliminate the perception and presence of hidden motives and agendas. It takes a while for people to learn that a good question is an opportunity to open up rather than a warning to run for cover.

Not "Why," but "What"

Changing "why" to "what" can reduce anxiety and intimidation. In one of the early versions of the four questions, the second question read, "*Why* is this happening this way?" The wording is normal and natural. Indeed, the question gets at why things are happening as they are. However, "why" questions tend to stir up a defensive response in people.

A colleague from the counseling department, Dr. Doug Little, pointed out that asking why implies a search for blame. As children, we remember the why questions: "Why isn't your homework done" or "Why is your room such a mess?" As adults, "Why is the report late" or "Why are you over budget?" conjure up the same emotional reactions.

The question is transformed by replacing *why* is it happening with *what* is causing it to happen this way. For example, "What is causing reports to be late," or "What is causing the department to be over budget?"

Now, the question is a search for understanding. In everyday conversations, particularly in the workplace, people fail to distinguish between arguing and asking. Asking why can come across as intimidating, evoking a defensive response. This is the beginning of an argument.

Douglas Stone, Bruce Patton, and Sheila Heen studied confrontational conversations. They found that ninety percent of the time, these conversations are arguing for a point or position. Only ten percent of the conversations involve seeking to understand. (See, *Difficult Conversations*, Viking Penguin 2000)

Asking why can be confrontational. It can abort the birth of mutual understanding and new insight. Learn to ask, "What is causing it to happen this way?" Reduce the level of fear and intimidation and you open the door to better solutions.

Create Shared Solutions

The snow glistened beyond the glass walls of the lodge. A fireplace in the center of the room was the focal point for the executive team. This event was the culmination of a series of planning sessions. Satisfaction rested on the group like a warm blanket. They shared the experience of a job well done.

Several weeks earlier we had had our first meeting together. My task was to establish a foundation of healthy relationships upon which the team could search for a better solution. I led them in a simple exercise of expressing mutual appreciation and support. These dedicated and well-meaning people risked being real.

The team's leader also needed to be on board. In the past, he was known for occasional angry and intimidating outbursts. However, he expressed a desire to work with the team to find a better answer. His heartfelt words were accepted by the team members as sincere. The search for a better solution was underway.

Each person tackled the hard work of gathering facts as together they answered the question, What's happening? Grappling with what was causing it to happen that way challenged authenticity at a personal and group level. They passed the test: The team searched for understanding rather than defending personal opinions and positions.

They created a clear statement of purpose supported by shared core values; it expressed what they had learned. Goals and action steps outlined what we will do next. Now, for a few moments, the team savored the fire, the sparkle in the snow, and their solution to a tough problem.

Their solution was born in the safety of healthy team relationships. Healthy relationships were also required to carry out the solution. Yet, this was not to be the case.

Three months later, the team and the organization found themselves in turmoil.

Poisonous Reactions

Carrying out the shared solution, the practical wisdom discovered by the group, was poisoned through venomous attacks, angry outbursts, and inquisitions designed to intimidate. In this case, the source of the toxin was the chief executive officer spewing out commands and ridiculing subordinates.

Shared wisdom burrowed underground in a frantic attempt to avoid the scramble for professional survival. Vicious words and decisions gunned down values and goals. The CEO's management by intimidation set the organization back a half decade.

What happened? Under stress, the stress of a financial crisis, the CEO reverted to his most familiar pattern of behavior, leadership through intimidation. In this extreme example, threats, bullying, and coercion chased off the best talent and destroyed the energy and creativity desperately needed in the organization. If you lead through intimidation, the *four questions* will not work.

The wise man doesn't give the right answers, he poses the right questions.

—Claude Levi-Strauss

CHAPTER 8

The Questions Are Empowering

The questions will work wonder and magic, if the relationships are safe enough to risk being real. If people sense intimidation, control, or blame, the questions will not function. If people sense acceptance, empathy, and understanding, the questions will open wonderful discussions that lead to learning, cooperation, united action and mutual success.

Leo Tolstoy wrote a fable called "The Three Questions." It once occurred to a certain king, that if he always knew the right time to begin everything, if he knew who the right people were and, above all, if he always knew the most important thing to do, he would never fail at anything he attempted.

The king searched for the answer to these three great questions:

When is the right time to begin?
Who are the right people to work with?
What is the most important thing to do?

The answers from across the kingdom were contradictory. Confusion reigned in the mind of the king. In the midst of his search, the king happened upon a man in need and gave him help. However, the king did not know the man was an enemy until after the help was given.

In the experience of helping an enemy, coupled with the counsel of an old man, the king discovered his answers: The right time is now. The most important person is the one I am with. And the greatest pursuit is to do good for that person.

The best time is now.
The most important person is you.
The greatest pursuit is your good.

These are the factors that make it safe enough for people to risk being real. A sense of psychological safety emerges in the presence of a person who is authentically focused on your good. In a healthy relationship, a safe relationship, you are more likely to risk being real. You are more likely to find the courage to tackle the problem. Leo Tolstoy's fable of "The Three Questions" offers an invitation to open up and be genuine.

There is one more factor that encourages people to risk being real. To the three questions in the fable, I would add a fourth: What is the most valuable discovery? The answer:
The most valuable discover is your true and best self.
When you are true to what is best about you, you help others risk being true to their best. When this is your purpose, the questions work like magic.

Empowering Relationships

You become a safe person for others when you risk being real. You are a safe person when you demonstrate to others by your words and actions, "The time we invest on this issue is important. You are essential to a successful outcome. I want what is good for you. I am confident that the wise answer comes from your true and best self."

WHEN RELATIONSHIPS ARE HEALTHY:
The questions will empower authenticity and effectiveness.

- *What is happening?* People are open to facts and feelings, attitudes and intuitions. You can put everything on the table—the good, the bad, and the ugly.
- *What is causing it to happen this way?* A search for deeper dynamics and helpful insights takes over. Individuals will accept their part of the responsibility.
- *What can we learn?* Learning is both personal and professional, for individuals and for the group. Creative discoveries made in this manner often have lasting impact.
- *What will we do next?* For groups, it is often united strategy and action that emerges from the discussion. Individuals come away with greater confidence as they determine to take the next step.

A safe, healthy relationship is essential for the questions to function. In healthy relationships, personal boundaries are respected, empathy is genuine, and appropriate transparency is exercised. People sense they are valued and validated.

A "Human Moment"

It isn't magic after all. It is what Edward Hallowell, writing in *Harvard Business Review*, called, "a human moment." It is a moment when you are paying attention, physically, emotionally, and intellectually. Hallowell defines his term:

> A human moment does not have to be draining or personally revealing. . . . A five-minute conversation can be a perfectly meaningful human moment. To make it work, you have to set aside what you are doing, put down the memo you were reading, disengage from your laptop, abandon your daydream, and focus on the person you're with. (*Harvard Business Review*, "The Human Moment at Work," January-February, 1999.)

Often, in a safe human moment, you can guide someone through the four questions in five minutes and help them unearth the treasured answer they need. On many occasions I have asked an administrative assistant or colleague to "help me think this through."

I tell them what I see happening and ask if they have other information or any sense of intuition to add. Then, we start looking at underlying causes. When the insight comes, learning and action follow naturally. Small daily problems can be frustrating and at times daunting. A little time with a safe person in a human moment can help you walk away with confidence in what to do next.

Other problems are more profound and personal. Pain is a fact of life; family life, organizational life, and church life. Divorce, mergers, and splits result in broken families, lost jobs, and shaken faith.

The experience of pain is normal. The healthy response is, "I will not waste pain, but learn and become a better person because of it." Hurtful experience can open the door to greater opportunities. You become a more authentic human being.

However, pain can become toxic. The hurtful experience can become a source of poison for the rest of your life. How the pain is handled determines the long-term effects.

Meeting with a safe person in a series of human moments as you explore the four questions will help process pain in a healthy way. It will take time; perhaps months. Healing will come. You cannot force your heart. You have to be ready.

When the time is right and your heart is prepared, the questions provide a way to make sense of what has happened. They help you dig deep into your own reservoir of inner wisdom. The questions guide you as you get on with your life.

Make Home a Safe Place

Guiding grown children is a new challenge for me. Between us, Shirley and I have five children, all within five years in age. They call from their cell phones. Sometimes they just want to talk, and sometimes they want help solving a problem:

"I have a tough meeting this morning; what do I say?"
"My boyfriend is with me. Counsel us."
"The professor is unjust, what should I do?"
"I want my life to make a difference."

On occasion, the questions need clear and direct answers. But, more often the conversations center on deep issues that carry emotions, values, and ambiguities. Rather than quick reactions, the solutions require courage, self-understanding, and personal control. Answers must be discovered rather than dictated.

This is not an easy world for kind people of principles and values. It is especially difficult for young adults to find their way. The worn paths of previous generations are concealed under a maze of uncertainty. They need practical wisdom.

Shirley and I want our home to be a safe place for our children. Home is where the door is always open for you, no matter what. Home is where you are out of harm's way. Home is where you can search your heart and soul, reconnect with your inner wisdom, and gather the courage you need to see it through.

You can be a safe person. You can "open your door," and provide a few moments "out of harm's way." Often, a human moment can make the difference for someone in your office. It can make the difference for someone in your family as well. In the safe harbor, authentic struggles can lead to effective solutions.

One of the reasons people stop learning is that they become less and less willing to risk failure.

—John W. Gardner

CHAPTER 9

Risk Being Real

Take a risk. You don't have to be "the one with all the answers." Give up fixing everyone else's problems. You don't have to solve everything all the time. You know the old adage, "Give a person a fish and there is food for a day; teach a person to fish and there is food for a lifetime." If you are willing to risk being real, the four questions open great possibilities for you:

- You will teach your children to make better decisions.
- You will solve problems with your marriage partner.
- You will develop the people you work with.
- You will help someone face a new challenge.
- You will guide a friend through a rough time.
- You will improve relationships at home and at work.
- You will become a more authentic person.

You can make a difference in the lives of others while growing personally and professionally. You can be a safe person who engages human moments as you ask four questions: What is happening? What is causing it to happen that way? What can you learn? What will you do next?

Be a Safe Person

Ambiguity is experiencing two conflicting feelings at the same time. Using the questions creates ambiguity. People desire to learn and yet, at the same moment, they are afraid to learn.

The desire to learn is natural. Every human being is born with it. In my doctoral work in education administration, I invested many hours of classroom study in leadership, organizational dynamics, and theories of learning. In addition to these studies, I was required to choose an inside minor. I chose to study how young children learn.

I learned that you don't have to teach little children so much as stay out of their way when they are learning. The desire to learn is overwhelming in young children. On the one hand, you must make sure they are not bored. On the other, the level of frustration must be tolerable. In the place between boredom and frustration, children learn.

Because you are a human being, the desire to learn follows you throughout your life. As an adult, frustration and boredom will hamper learning. Yet, there is another factor that impacts adult learners. Adults are often afraid of learning.

As adults, we discover that learning something new may result in a period of appearing incompetent, being rejected by others, or being punished by those in authority over you. Golfers know that learning a new swing results in worse scores for awhile.

When you are learning a new golf swing, you look as if you don't know what you are doing. Friends tease and belittle in good fun. You have to buy everyone's lunch at the nineteenth hole. Appearing incompetent and being rejected and punished are part and parcel to most learning experiences for adults.

The stakes increase when you move from the golf course to your work and your home. A man may have a real desire to learn to be a better husband. A staff member may want to develop a new competency. A boss may long to figure out how she is part of the problem so that she can become part of the solution. Yet, fear may stop their progress.

Increase the Desire to Learn

The desire to learn may be buried under the fear of appearing incompetent, being rejected, or being punished. To create an environment in which adults are encouraged to learn, you must adhere to two principles:

> *First, the desire to learn must be*
> *greater than the fear of learning.*
> Second, lowering the fear of learning
> increases the desire to learn.

A safe person does just that. A safe person lowers your fear of learning because you know he or she has your best interest at heart. There is no hidden agenda, maneuvering, or manipulation. A safe person simply wants what is best for you.

You become a safe person when you are authentic, when you are true to your best self. Your words and actions demonstrate that you are genuine:

The best time is now
The most important person is you
The greatest pursuit is your good
The most valuable discovery is your true and best self

You need safe people in your life. You can be a safe person for others. Mutual trust and respect are hallmarks of healthy relationships. However, if distrust and fear dominate the relationship, the four questions are not as effective. For example, you help create safe relationships when accountability is a mean of mutual success rather than primarily "holding feet to the fire."

The four questions work in a wide variety of situations that share a common element: *The most valuable answer is under the surface.* To explore under the surface is to risk being real. You can help people when you determine to:

Be a Safe Person;
Enter a Human Moment;
Apply the four questions.

As you learn to use the questions, it will seem awkward at first. If it feels odd and stilted when you first use the questions, it means you are on the right track. Keep at it and you will be effective. The questions will become a habit that will help you as you continue on your life's journey. Your personal experience will be transformed into new insight and valuable wisdom.

Internalize the four questions

Here is a practical way to begin: use the four questions as a daily outline in your personal journal for the next thirty days. Answer each question. Determine to learn one lesson each day for the next month.

- *What happened?* Focus on one event that took place today. Look at the outside and inside of the experience. Note what you saw and what you did. Tune in to what you thought and felt.
- *What caused it to happen that way?* Look over the details. Also, look at the big picture. Examine the facts. Follow your hunches. When you find an answer to question 2, push yourself a little deeper by asking, "And, what else?"
- *What can I learn?* Use your head and your heart. There is logical wisdom and wisdom that logic can't explain. Answer question 3 by imagining that you are explaining what you learned to another person.
- *What will I do next?* Apply the lesson you have learned. You may find an application that is a single action or a new plan. It may be an application that prepares you for another event or opens you to another option.

Following this pattern for thirty days will help you learn to use the questions. You will discover, personally, the power of the questions. You will also develop skill and insight you will use as you guide others through the questions.

Education should be the process of helping everyone discover his or her uniqueness.

—Leo Buscaglia

CHAPTER 10

Make it a Habit

As a parent, marriage partner, teacher, minister, team leader, board member, or friend, you will find that learning to use the questions regularly will reap great rewards.

Your relationships will deepen. Learning to employ the questions will enrich your communication skills. Helping people make positive discoveries builds bonds in your family, on the job, and in all the relationships in your life.

Your understanding will improve. Exploring causes and dynamics will expand your understanding and help you to be more flexible and adaptable. Over time, you will cultivate better perception and insight into diverse situations and problems.

Your wisdom will mature. The best learning is from experience: your own experience and the experience of others. Consistently asking the questions will put you squarely on a path that will develop your judgment as well as your appreciation for the complexity of life.

Your actions will be more focused. Many people who find themselves in a crisis scramble for the quickest way out. The result can be a move from frying pan to fire. The persistent use of the questions will sharpen your solutions, direct your actions, and create more positive results.

You authenticity will increase. There are people in your life who take control by telling you who you are and setting your limitations. You seize your own life when you learn to validate your true and best self. The questions will help you discover, confirm, and strengthen your authenticity.

Make it a Routine

Implement a pattern of using the four questions regularly. Make it a routine and it will become a habit that leads to a more fulfilling life.

FIRST, ask yourself the questions. Ask them when you face a problem or new challenge. Make it a habit to ask yourself the questions when you succeed and when you don't. With consistent use, the questions will form a pattern in your thinking. You will go through them without realizing it.

To remind yourself, carry one of the wallet sized four questions cards found at the back of this book. Use the questions thirty times in the next month. You will give birth to a habit.

Habits are born out of repetition.
Habits are born out of repetition.
Habits are born out of repetition.
Habits are born out of repetition.
Habits are born out of repetition.

SECOND, practice the questions with friends and family. The questions have the potential to transform relationships in your home and with your friends. Tell them you are learning to ask the questions. Ask if they would be willing to help you.

It will require only a few attempts and your confidence will grow. You will learn to ask the questions with different words and in different forms while maintaining the flow and integrity of the questions. Soon, you will be great at it. It will feel odd at first, but keep it up. It works.

THIRD, implement the questions at work. This may take a change in atmosphere. The questions require a human moment, a time when you pay attention physically, emotionally, and intellectually. They will not work in a fear-filled moment when intimidation, blame, and control are prowling about. Be a safe person and people will risk being real around you.

Start using the questions at work by asking others to help you think through an issue. Use your four questions card. Explain that the questions don't make problems go away or solutions appear with ease. The questions work because you are willing to work at it.

Empowering Accountability

In all organizations, businesses, churches, or groups of volunteers, people need someone to take their report and help them solve problems. Make the questions a routine and rewards will follow.

A business owner heard this idea in a seminar I presented. He took it to heart and put it into practice. He told me he was meeting with each of his staff members, individually, every week. Their reports contained actions and results. The conversations followed the four questions:

- *What has happened?* Actions and achievements are reported. The results can be positive or negative. Usually it is a combination of both.
- *What is causing it to happen that way?* If the results are primarily positive, it's an opportunity to explore what works, and reinforce positive action. If the results are negative, it's an opportunity to give feedback, correct errors, solve problems, and make decisions.
- *What can you learn?* In the face of complex issues, self discovered solutions are most often better than handing down orders. When a person has a personal "ah-ha" moment, the learning is more likely to lead toward lasting improvement.
- *What will you do next?* The action plan may need to change. Goals may need to be modified. Taking care of distractions and other demands may be the wise thing to do. Staff members are empowered when they are involved in choosing what to do next.

Start now. Learn to use the questions. Turn them into a routine. They will become a habit, a way of thinking that will help you help others.

Help Me Solve My Problems

After several months of work, the ministerial team came to a crisis moment. I was serving as an outside consultant. The team had tackled several large challenges together. They were ready for a new level of authenticity. The senior pastor conveyed his heart to them, "I want to help. I want to be a better support for you. What can I do?"

Silence fell around the table. In a moment of vulnerable self-disclosure, a team member said to the senior pastor, "When I am struggling with a problem, you tend to take the problem away from me and solve it yourself. I believe you think this helps. It doesn't. If you really want to help, don't solve my problems for me; help me solve my problems."

As you learn to help others solve their own problems, you will become a better parent, a more empowering leader, a more compassionate minister, and a true friend. You will become more genuine, open to the wisdom in others, and in tune with your own inner wisdom.

The "silly" question is the first intimation of some totally new development.
—Alfred North Whitehead

C H A P T E R **11**

When to Use the Four Questions

On the following pages are ten different situations in which you can use the four questions. All of them have a common element: The most valuable answer is under the surface. The process for using the questions is the same in each case: 1) be a safe person, 2) enter a human relationship, 3) apply the four questions.

Use the questions to repeat your successes.

Don't ask me no questions and I won't tell you no lies.
—Lynyrd Skynyrd

When something goes right, you may grab at a surface explanation and miss deeper understanding. However, your competency will improve if you dig underneath what has happened and think through all that caused your success. Look at structures and systems as well as personal actions. When you learn the key elements of getting it right and reaching your goal, you are more likely to do it again.

Use the questions to figure out what went wrong.

The answer, my friend, is blowin' in the wind.
—Peter, Paul and Mary

Regrets are neither "my entire fault," nor "their entire fault." The truth is more complex. You will learn more from your regrets than your successes. Exploring regrets requires a safe person. Confidentiality and personal integrity are essential. It takes a special person to provide the safety needed to dig the wisdom out of a regretful experience. If the regret is particularly painful and personal, there will be several levels of wisdom to unearth.

Use the questions to solve a problem.

These questions are too deep for such a simple man.
—Supertramp

A tough problem can leave you frustrated and bored. Both experiences will halt learning. Remember to keep your focus on the main issue. Break open the problem by gathering more information about what is happening. Then, search for cause rather than blame. Look for the patterns, the structures, systems, or dynamics underneath the situation. You are on your way to a new solution.

Use the questions to lead team decision making.

The answer lies within, so why not take a look.
—Cat Stevens

"Participative Decision Making" is touted by leadership and organizational experts. The four questions provide a practical way to proceed. You are a safe person when you genuinely and appropriately state your view and demonstrate your openness to the view of others. Let everyone speak. List all the information. Let the team dig out the causes and dynamics, structures and systems, attitudes and motives that are driving the issue.

Use the questions to make a presentation.

The answers are getting harder and harder and there ain't no way to bargain or barter.

—Blues Travler

The questions are an excellent outline. Think through the questions as preparation for your presentation. Outline your speech: 1) This is what's happening now; 2) These are the reasons causing it to happen this way; 3) This is what we must learn, and 4) Here is the challenge of what we will do next. This is a simple way to present information that leads to action.

Use the questions to get started on a new challenge.

There's more than one answer to these questions.

—The Indigo Girls

The first day of a new job or receiving a new assignment can be daunting. Where do you begin? You want to appear competent and effective; but don't let appearances fool you. The questions get you started in the right direction. You need to learn, and learn fast. Investigate what is happening. Talk to people. Read all you can. Keep track of what you discover. In time, patterns and dynamics will appear. Then, your real learning begins.

Use the questions to work through conflict.

Why do we never get an answer when we're knocking on the door?

—The Moody Blues

Most people avoid conflict, often at a heavy cost to their relationships, peace of mind, and career advancement. Even when conflict results in creative solutions, it is not fun. Conflict is inevitable. It is a moment of testing. The questions are a means of conflict resolution. Risk being real. Everyone has something at stake. What do you have at stake in the conflict?

Use the questions in an interview.

The question to everyone's answer is usually asked from within.

—The Steve Miller Band

The best interviews are not a collection of loaded questions such as, "Do you like to work with people?" or "What is your greatest weakness?" Good interviews encourage people to tell stories of personal success and regret; "Tell me about a time when . . ." Use the questions to guide people through their stories. Use follow-up questions such as "and then what?"

and "what else?" to demonstrate your interest and uncover deeper insights.

Use the questions to develop others.

There's no reply at all.

—Genesis

Helping others expand their potential, gain new skills, overcome setbacks, unravel problems, and be their best is your role in many situations. As a parent, spouse, supervisor, mentor, minister, coach, or friend, you can help others grow. Use the questions routinely. Allow and encourage each person to find their own answers. You can use the questions to help them dig below the surface, discover their dream and realize their potential.

Use the questions to become a more authentic person.

How can we have wondered about so much for so long and received so few answers.

—The Judybats

When you live on the surface, life becomes a shallow scramble to look effective and get by. Even great financial success or career advancement will become hollow and empty. There is more to you and more to life. Dig down deep. Learn to think. Bring your best and true self to your work and your home. Be a safe person, enter "human moments," and apply four questions: What is happening? What is causing it to happen this way? What can I learn? What will I do next?

A change in growth takes place when a person has risked himself and dares to become involved with experimenting with his how life.

—Herbert Otto

CHAPTER 12

You Can Empower People

As you use the *four questions*, you will discover better ways to solve problems, advance your thinking skills, and develop a greater repertoire of behaviors that will improve your relationships. You will increase your ability to empower others by helping them discover their own answers and solutions.

Don is a great business leader and also coaches in a Junior Basketball league. The boys are between ten and twelve years of age. One Saturday, the team made a particularly poor showing. Don, who was learning the *four questions*, guided the boys to a moment of team discovery.

- **What happened?** The boys quickly regurgitated the flaws and foibles of the game. Everyone had a story to tell. Don carefully listened to everyone's tail.
- **What caused it to happen that way?** Everyone had an interpretation to share. Don provided the structure needed to move past blame and faultfinding.

What ever cause was suggested by one of the boys, Don would ask, "And, what else?"

- **What did you learn?** The motivation to be a winning team kicked the boys thinking into gear. They learned that each one of them had something to learn.
- **What will you do next?** This was the moment of commitment. The boys asked for a review of basic skills. They challenged each other to play as a team. They also wanted to double their determination to be the best.

Could a coach want more? Don knew that this was what they needed. He could have declared his intentions and delivered the needed practice routines without consulting the boys. However, when the boys made the discovery themselves, motivation and cooperation soared. And, by learning to solve the problem together, they were a better team.

You can learn to help others discover their own solutions and answers. This skill will make you a better parent, coach, manager, teacher, or leader. The questions are empowering. This chapter is filled with practical suggestions for putting the questions to work.

When you ask, "What happened?"

Ask this question with *compassion*. The person you are asking is asking themselves a question, "Why do you want to know?" It takes a healthy relationship to work through the questions together. Begin with interest and empathy, not advice.

Everyone has a story to tell. However, you rarely have the opportunity to tell your whole story without being interrupted, corrected, advised, or ignored. By demonstrating your genuine concern and understanding, you help others relive their experience. This is where the path toward inner wisdom begins.

Help them recall the inward experience and the outward event. Often a person will tell a bit of their story and wait to see if you are truly engaged and paying attention. Keep asking, "What else?" These two words, asked with authenticity, express interest. Here are other ways to ask, "What else?"

- What happened next?
- What were you thinking/feeling when that happened?
- What did you think/hope/fear would happen?
- What has happened since then?

As you coach people through this part of the process, two things need to happen. First, *establish trust and respect.* You should tune in to what they are feeling and respond appropriately, take an active interest in their concerns and needs, and listen with openness and understanding.

Second, *engage their motivation.* They may be motivated to complain, explain, defend, or dodge issues and events. You stir the motivation to learn when you connect with their experience, validate their experience, and identify with the internal conflict and uncertainty they are currently experiencing.

You know it is time to move to the next question when the experience has been fully aired, their inquisitive interest has been ignited; and they are more objective and reflective.

When you ask, "What caused it to happen that way?"

Commitment is put to the test with this question. It is encouraging to tell your story; it is challenging to dig for root causes. Your good character is essential to keep this part of the process productive. Check your own agenda. What is at stake for you?

Human beings attach interpretation to all important events. In fact, your first interpretation colors the way you remember the event. The journey toward inner wisdom demands a commitment to set aside pre-conceived notions and genuinely look for new insights and understanding.

Again, the two word question works, "What else?" At this point you don't want to challenge the causes that are offered. You want to help people explore other causes as they search for the root causes. Provide enough structure to encourage the flow of insight. A simple way to do this is to write down each "cause" as it is given. Then ask, "What else?" Also consider these questions:

- What are the unspoken thoughts/hopes/fears?
- What are the unexpressed needs or interests?
- What are the conflicting needs or forces?
- What is personally significant about this to you?

Your challenge at this point is, first, to embrace the process and second, search for truth. You will help others *embrace the process* when you provide supportive accountability, personal encouragement and reflection, and manage the process for them.

The *search for truth* rests upon mutual trust and respect. Provide feedback, address concerns, and probe the strengths and gaps in their thinking. Challenge them to assess the validity of their interpretation of the event.

Searching for root causes is challenging. People discover truth in different ways. Some approach the search through cold logic. They weigh and consider the evidence. Others find truth in stories about other people. The stories are like a ray of light on the path.

Another way that people search for truth is measuring conduct and choices against a standard or code that they follow faithfully. Finally, there are people who are deeply sensitive to human complexity. They do not see life as either/or, but as both/and.

When the search for true root causes is particularly difficult, a person needs a quiet time, a safe place and a special friend. You can be the friend they need. They need you to be a friend who speaks the truth and keeps promises.

You know it is time to move to the third question when the individual or group has been attentive and receptive to input from others, thoughtfully considered a variety of perspectives, and embraced fresh insight.

When you ask, "What can you learn?"

Confidence is the escort of learning. The quality of work invested in discovering root causes paves the way for new learning. Root causes are often (but not always) objective dynamics buried in the situation. However, learning is always personal. You can search for root cause with a commitment to principles. To learn requires confidence in your sense of purpose.

The key to learning is personal values and vision. When you connect values and vision to need learning, you release determination and self-discipline. Lasting change must be rooted in core beliefs, personal passion, clear focus and authentic action. Inner confidence is the companion of deep learning.

You help people articulate and internalize what they have learned from experience with two words, "What if . . ." The two words shift the focus from past to future. They move the emphasis from postmortem to prediction. With this shift, new learning can be tied to personal mission, service to others, and faithfulness to core beliefs.

Ask, "What can you learn from this experience?" When you hear the answer, respond with, "What if you applied that at home?" or "What if you shared that insight with your team?" or "What if you learned to make that a habit?" The possibilities are limitless.

Your goal is to *ignite positive energy* as new learning is connected to personal vision and values. You also *encourage focused results* by generating goals, targets and projects that apply the new learning. It is time to move to the final question when the lessons are personalized, the energy is high, and application is clear.

When you ask, "What will you do next?"

Courage leads to action. To act out of courage is self-empowering. And, to change as a result of new insight and learning takes courage. Courage is like a kite on the wind;

it needs a string to remain grounded. That's your task in this final step. As the guide or coach in the process, the person or group you are working with needs your mature wisdom.

Your task is to *provide strategic wisdom*. Help them plan action steps, set timelines, and secure resources. Also, *provide empowering accountability*. Set a time when you will listen to their report and help them solve problems.

Quality questions create a quality life. Successful people ask better questions, and as a result, they get a better life.

—Anthony Robbins

A Fable:

Questions at the Crossroads

Once upon a time, **IT** happened. **IT** was an Involved Tangle of Increasing Trouble. There **IT** lay, at the place where paths crossed.

From four directions, four strangers stumbled upon **IT** at the same moment. The first arrived from the North. His name was *THAT'S INTERESTING*. *THAT WORKS* and *THAT'S RIGHT* journeyed from the East and South respectively. And *THAT'S COURAGEOUS* arrived from the West. Each stranger decided that he alone could best solve **IT**.

The first stranger, *THAT'S INTERESTING*, preferred looking at things from another way. He asked lots of questions and concluded that **IT** was full of Irresponsible Tangents that would be appealing to explore.

THAT WORKS did not agree. He believed that they should consider what is readily known and select a solution that seems practical. He was confident that they must Impose a Time limit for solving **IT**.

His assurance troubled *THAT'S RIGHT*. He was skeptical of quick, new solutions. He wanted the right answer, and preferred what's been tested and proven. The Importance of Truth is the way to solve **IT**.

THAT'S COURAGEOUS had been listening. He was frustrated with all the answers. He wanted action. he believed that solving **IT** required Implementing Tactics and then see what happens.

At this, a great conflict arose among the four strangers. The argument continued for two days and nights. Each made his point, belittled the others and retreated into his Individual way of Thinking. All this time, **IT** was growing larger and more difficult to deal with. The strangers were Increasingly Testy and Internally Touchy.

When the sun rose on the third day, a blind man stood with the four strangers. The four strangers appointed the blind man as judge. The blind man agreed to hear each case and decide the best way to solve **IT**.

THAT'S COURAGEOUS spoke with boldness, "We need to do something, whatever it is." A low scoff came from *THAT'S RIGHT*, "We need to find someone to blame." *THAT WORKS* was frantic, "We need to find a quick fix, right now." Nervously, *THAT'S INTERESTING*, offered, "We need to take more time to think before we decide."

At noon, the blind man silenced the four strangers. In the quiet, he recalled a story from another time and place:

80

A Fable: Questions at the Crossroads

There was once a group of blind men who stumbled upon an elephant. Since none of the blind men had ever seen an elephant, they didn't know what to make of it. Each touched the elephant. One said it was a wall, because he had touched the elephant's side. Another felt the leg of the elephant and declared that it was a tree. A third was certain it was a rope, for he had grabbed the tail. The fourth, clutching to the elephants wiggling trunk, was convinced it was a great snake.

Turning to the four strangers, the sightless seer inquired, "Which blind man saw the elephant?"

The four strangers sat motionless. Each realized he could see part of the picture. And, each realized he had a blind spot.

THAT'S INTERESTING was good at surveying the situation from many perspectives, but had difficulty making a decision. He turned to the group and acknowledged, "I'm best at taking the initiative by asking ***"What's happening?"***

THAT'S RIGHT had a passion for discovering the root of things, but did not like to implement change. He confessed, "I should confine myself to discovering, ***"What's causing it to happen that way?"***

THAT WORKS had a talent for summarizing what is known, but was easily tempted to take the first answer rather than wait for the best one. He knew his place, "I use what the two of you accomplish to figure out, ***"What can we learn?"***

THAT'S COURAGEOUS was daring and ready to take a risk, but did not think about consequences. "I understand now," he said with resolve, "I'll wait until all three of you are finished. Then, implementing all your work, I'll answer the question, *"What will we do next?"*

The four strangers shook hands at the place where roads intersect. They were strangers no more. They were partners. And, the blind man pointed at **IT**. To the amazement of the strangers, the problem was gone. In the place where paths cross was a better answer. The strangers conquered **IT** by combining Individual Talents to uncover Incredible Treasure.

Language was invented to ask questions. Answers may be given by grunts and gestures, but questions must be spoken. Humanness came of age when human beings asked the first question. Social stagnation results not from a lack of answers but from the absence of the impulse to ask questions.

—Eric Hoffer

T-N-T Discussions

T-N-T means *Think-N-Talk, Talk-N-Think.* You will learn more when you invest time in discussing and reflecting (talking and thinking) on the concepts presented in this book. Exchanging ideas, insights, and responses with another person or group will greatly enrich your understanding and skill with the four questions.

On the following pages are three discussions that employ the questions. The discussions will help you practice the questions. The discussions are designed to be used by such diverse groups as work teams, office staff, church boards, marriage partners, friends, study groups, or accountability partners. You will also find the discussions helpful if you use them alone.

T-N-T Discussion #1–Learn from Experience

Read chapters 1, 2, and 3.

1. What ideas from the first three chapters were most helpful to you?
2. Share a personal experience that taught you a valuable lesson in life. Share your experience by answering the four questions:

   - *What happened? Describe* what you experienced; the facts, feelings, intuitions, etc.
   - *What caused it to happen that way? Explain* the dynamics, motives, patterns, etc. underneath what caused it to happen that way.
   - *What did I learn? Share* the principles, truth, "common sense," practical wisdom, etc., you learned from your experience.
   - *What did I do next? Tell* how you apply the lessons you learned from your experience.

3. What is the key idea you will take away from this discussion?

T-N-T Discussion #2–Work Together

Read chapters 4, 5, and 6.

1. What ideas from the chapters 4, 5, and 6 were most helpful to you?
2. Explore a recent experience you share as a group or team (or individual, if you are using the questions for personal reflection). Uncover the lessons in the experience by working together to answer the four questions:

   - **What happened?** *Describe* what you as a group or team experienced; Look at the "outside" and "inside" of the experience. Note what was said and done as well as individual thoughts and emotions.
   - **What caused it to happen that way?** *Explain* the dynamics, motives, patterns, etc. underneath what caused it to happen that way. Look at the "trees" and the "forest."
   - **What did I learn?** *Uncover* the principles, truth, common sense, practical wisdom, etc., you learned from the experience. Lessons come "head first" and "heart first."
   - **What did I do next?** *Determine* how you could apply the lessons you learned together. Consider "finishers" and "starters." Look at plans and options.

3. What is the key idea you will take away from this discussion?

T-N-T Discussion #3–Toxic Relationships

Read chapter 7.

1. What ideas from chapter 7 were most helpful to you? What experiences come to mind?

2. Explore the power of toxic relationships. Draw on the variety of personal experiences in the group (or as an individual). Think about toxic friendships, workplaces, family relationships, etc. Pool your knowledge and combine your answers to the four questions as you seek a deeper understanding of toxic relationships.

   - *What happens* when relationships are toxic? List at least twenty *results* of toxic relationships. Include facts, emotions, symptoms, outcomes, problems, etc. Remember, describe what happens when relationships are toxic.

   - *What causes it to happen that way* (when relationships are toxic)? List at least ten underlying *dynamics*. Describe what causes toxic relationships to produce the *results* listed above.

   - *What have you learned* about toxic relationships? List at least five lessons of *practical wisdom* you could teach others about toxic relationships. Describe how to deal with the *dynamics* of toxic relationships listed above.

   - *What will you do next* time you must deal with a toxic relationship? List at least three actions. Describe how to apply the lessons of *practical wisdom* listed above.

3. What is the key idea you will take away from this discussion?

T-N-T Discussion #4—Safe People

Read chapter 8.

1. What ideas in this chapter was most helpful to you? Share a practical example from your experience.
2. When considering what it means to be a safe person (or a safe group of people), you have a great deal of practical wisdom. What is it? To get in touch with the practical wisdom of your group or team, answer the four questions.

   - *What is happening* that indicates we are a safe group (a safe person)? List the *results* of being part of this safe group and with these safe people.
   - *What is causing it to happen that way* (what makes our group safe)? List the *dynamics* that make your group (or you) safe enough for others to risk being real.
   - *What can you learn* about being a safe person or group? List the *practical wisdom* you could share with other groups or persons who want to provide a safe place to be real.
   - *What will you do next* to maintain or increase the sense of safety? List *actions and attitudes* that will maintain or improve the safety of your group.

3. What is the key idea you will take away from this discussion?

T-N-T Discussion #5–Get Personal

Read chapters 8 and 9.

1. What ideas in these chapters were helpful to you? Share a practical example from your experience.
2. Use the *four questions* to find a solution to a current problem or challenge. This may be a personal or professional issue. Keep a few notes that record your thinking process.

   - *What happened?*
   - *What caused it to happen that way?*
   - *What did I learn?*
   - *What will I do next?*

3. Each person will tell how they used the questions to deal with a current issue.
4. What did you learn from hearing how others use the *four questions*?

T-N-T Discussion #6–Empower Others

Read chapters 10, 11 and 12.

1. What ideas in these chapters were helpful to you? Share a practical example from your experience.
2. Guide someone else through the *four questions*. This may be a colleague, friend, or family member. Keep a few notes to help you recall the process.

   - *What happened?*
   - *What caused it to happen that way?*
   - *What did I learn?*
   - *What will I do next?*

3. Each person will tell how they guided another person through the questions. (Warning: Protect confidentiality! Ask the person for permission to share the experience with your group.)
4. What did you learn from hearing how others use the four questions to empower others?

About the Author

RICHARD LESLIE PARROTT, PH.D.

Dr. Parrott is the Founder and President of *Seize Your Life, Inc.,* whose purpose is to help individuals and organizations take hold of life's full potential by guiding them on a journey toward inner confidence, commitment, courage and compassion. The process helps individuals and organizations reach their goals through healthy relationships, good character, significant purpose and mature wisdom.

Dr. Parrott has served in professional leadership for thirty years. For six years he was the Director of a Doctoral Program at Ashland University and Assistant Professor of Leadership. He is also the founding Executive Director of the Sandberg Leadership Center at Ashland University, and had oversight of a million dollar Lilly grant on mentoring leaders. He has facilitated national roundtables and edited books on Leadership Character and Leadership and Power.

Dr. Parrott is the author of *Carpe Vitam: Seize Your Life; True and Best: Authentic Living, Better Answers to Tougher*

Questions and *Leadership Fundamentals*. He writes a monthly newsletter, "Worth Repeating," that is available in e-form.

His particular interest and expertise is personal and professional development. Richard is frequently called upon as a key note speaker and seminar leader. He has worked collaboratively with leadership centers at Yale, Claremont, and Gordon-Conwell. He has held seminars in strategic planning, team building, and leadership development for groups such as the State of Ohio Board of Pharmacy, the state wide Executive Board of the Chamber of Commerce, the Seattle Leadership Conference, and the Caucus of Republican Senators of the Ohio State Legislature.

Dr. Parrott has created and currently presents *The Balanced Leader*, a ten-seminar series for team leaders and managers and *Transformational Coaching*, a companion series for executive managers. The programs increase personal authenticity, improve professional competency, and impact business capacity. The next step in leadership development is *Leader to Leader*, a program that provides advanced leadership training and in-depth team assessments.

Dr. Parrott has also written a program for improving relationships Based on the Myers-Briggs Type Indicator (MBTI), Personalities @ Work Master Series is seven (7) sessions that introduce team members to "personality types," involves them in personal discovery, and provides group conversations on topics such as "Communication Problems," "Conflict," and "What works best for me." This program is currently used by business organizations and teams across the country.

Dr. Parrott and his wife, Shirley are a team. Shirley has been a Realtor for twenty years and was in the top one percent of all Realtors in the nation for nine consecutive years.

About the Author

Shirley and Richard are co-founders of *Seize Your Life, Inc.* They are fully committed to helping individuals and organizations take hold of life's full potential.

www.SeizeYourLife.com